|Foreword

The importance of protecting babies is a longstanding priority for the NSPCC and since the launch of the FULL STOP Campaign in 1999 we have run a number of awareness and public education initiatives addressing this key issue. We have also distributed thousands of copies of our leaflet *Handle with care*, aimed at parents, on the dangers of shaking and hitting babies. We are therefore pleased to be associated with the *Protecting babies' heads* toolbox by Lisa Coles and published by the Community Practitioners and Health Visitors Association. We believe that it will make an important contribution to the protection of babies.

The toolbox demonstrates the importance of prevention strategies. We know that many head injuries can be prevented. Too often parents are not aware of the fact that shaking babies and rough handling can be dangerous and that there are practical steps that they can take to ensure that their babies are not at risk. Sadly, many parents do not know what to do or where to go for support. Professionals have a key role to play.

The approach taken with this toolbox is special because while it is aimed at professionals and seeks to raise their awareness and improve their learning, it also contains practical advice, messages, and the template of a resource aimed at parents. If we are to influence parents' attitudes and behaviour so that they do not harm their babies' heads, it is important that we not only provide information but that this is also reinforced by the professionals who are working with them. Professionals have a key part to play in identifying vulnerable families, monitoring their progress, and providing support.

I hope that the toolbox will be widely used and that it will stimulate local discussions on what professionals can do to better safeguard babies.

Christopher Cloke
Head of Child Protection Awareness and Diversity
NSPCC

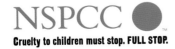

Acknowledgements

This document is written by Dr Lisa Coles and is based on research undertaken in the Department of Child Health, Wales College of Medicine, Cardiff University, Head of Department, Professor Jo Sibert, and Head of Community Section, Dr Alison Kemp. It has been supported by collaboration with Cardiff and Vale NHS Trust, Primary Care Directorate, Director Dianna Callaghan, endorsed and financially supported by the NSPCC and produced by the CPHVA.

The author gives grateful acknowledgement to Lynne Collins, health visitor, for research assistance and critical review.

Other colleagues in the trust, particularly Rev Beverley Smith, Head of Primary Care Nursing, and the health visitors who evaluated the toolbox, have contributed significantly. Thanks are also due to members of the Project Board, especially Dr Sally Holland, Lecturer, School of Social Sciences and Judy Cousins, Lecturer in Primary Care Nursing, School of Nursing and Midwifery, Cardiff University; Caroline Jones, Designated Child Protection Nurse, NPHS, S E Wales; Veronica Grant, Training and Consultancy Co-ordinator NSPCC and Sure Start staff.

Advice on clarity of wording for the teaching tool was given by Dr Lucy Coles, medical communications specialist, and from Mencap for the Parent Information sheet.

Funding for the original research was from The Nuffield Foundation, The Patrick Berthould Trust and The Children's Research Fund. Funding for the continuing prevention research programme was from The Welcome Trust, and currently, Child Safe Wales and Cerebra.

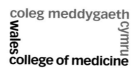
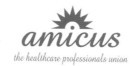
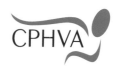

It is suggested that both child abuse and accidents are failures of carers to protect small children adequately. In abuse children are not protected from adult anger and in accidents they are not protected from dangerous environments[1]. Prevention must address both types of failure.

Contents of toolbox

The contents of this toolbox are a self directed learning tool for professional individual or group learning, references, internet resources and leaflets for use in practice.

There are colour coded boxes in the sections to assist learning. The Assessment Questions are for guided reading and self assessment. The answers are found in the text.

The two sections of the teaching tool are followed by two leaflets for photocopying and use in practice for preventing shaking and head injuries in babies. These are a Parent Information leaflet to be discussed with mothers and fathers and inserted into the Parent Held Child Health Record book, or similar, for future reference. The Practice Guide is for professionals as an aide-mémoire of the key points of the teaching tool. It can be carried in a Diary, or similar, as a reminder for use on home visits. These tools are tucked inside the back cover.

LEARNING OBJECTIVES

On completion of this self directed learning, professionals who work with small babies will be able to:
1   Understand how brain damage can occur in babies and its effects;
2   Understand the value and limitations of assessing risk;
3   Develop strategies to protect babies' heads.

STRUCTURE OF LEARNING TOOL
ASSESSMENT QUESTIONS
INFORMATION AND STRATEGIES
CASE EXAMPLES FROM RESEARCH.

Background and theory

1 | INTRODUCTION AND AIMS

This evidenced-based self learning tool is intended for use in preventing non-accidental head injury (NAHI), including shaking injuries, and accidental head injury in babies. It aims to provide a basis for developing early preventive measures for use in everyday practice. The tool has been reviewed by health visitors and a team of advisors.

In scope, this tool is not expected to prevent the most complex and violent of cases. It is aimed at the population of parents who might otherwise be ignored or progress to a more severe level of risk of injuring a baby's head. It raises awareness of the triggers and markers for such potential.

There is limited research on preventing head injuries in babies. This document refers to the research findings of the Severnside subdural haemorrhage study[2–6]. The tools for parents and practitioners, which are found after the references in Section 2, are influenced by ongoing research in which the views of mothers and fathers have been sought of the best way of approaching the prevention of head injuries.

The timeliness of this tool is reinforced by recent reports which stress the priorities of a culture of prevention, early interventions and providing a universal service to all families with new babies[7–10].

Defining prevention
Prevention, in the context of public health, is defined as reduction in the risk of a future adverse health event.
- Once injury to the brain has occurred there is no going back; prevention is paramount.
- Prevention includes macro level initiatives such as public awareness, policy and legal issues as well as interventions on the micro level of informing and educating.
- It is questionable whether risk can ever be eliminated in child protection work.

The toolbox aims to improve prevention and so lead to improved outcomes by reducing death, disability, behavioural and learning problems resulting from shaking and other injuries to babies' heads.

2 | INCIDENCE AND OUTCOMES

Non-accidental head injury
Among all types of child abuse, non-accidental head injury is the leading cause of death and long term disability.
- It is the most common cause of traumatic death in children under 1 year of age[11].
- Subdural haemorrhage (bleeding into the subdural space between the membranes that surround the brain) is a major manifestation of non-accidental head injury in babies, including shaking injuries.
- The UK national figures of non-accidental subdural haemorrhage reported in children under 12 months are in the order of 21–24 per 100,000 per year, rising to 36 per 100,000 children under 6 months old[12,13].

This equates to about 200 new hospital cases per year under 12 months of age compared with 187 Sudden Infant Deaths in England and Wales in 2002[14]. Despite traditional campaigns, cases of physical abuse, including fatal abuse, do not seem to be reducing[15].

In Wales, for example, statistics show
- Babies in Cardiff are at high risk of abusive head injury, including shaking injuries;[16]
- Children who are most at risk of severe physical abuse are infants under 12 months old where 54 per 100,000 per year sustain severe non-accidental injuries;
- In this age group the highest risk is in infants under 6 months of age[17].

Shaken baby syndrome
Non-accidental head injury is often referred to as shaken baby syndrome. This is defined as a young child who has been shaken violently with a whiplash effect on the bridging veins in the subdural space. Rotational and acceleration/deceleration forces are implied[18].
- The resultant subdural haemorrhage is seen on neuro-radiological imaging or at post mortem.
- Retinal haemorrhages (bleeding within the retina of the eye) may co-exist.
- There may be hypoxia (where the brain is deprived of oxygen).
- Impact injuries with skull fractures are not unknown.

There may be other injuries elsewhere on the body typical of physical child abuse, such as fractures and bruising[19,13].

Bruising and non-accidental head injury
Babies with fatal intracranial injury can be admitted to hospital with no external bruising.
- Bruises can fade quickly.
- Bruises may not have had time to appear.
- The skin may have been protected by clothing.
- It is speculated that the force used to grip around the chest under the arm pits may not be adequate to produce bruising.

However, bruises on the lower leg or ankle in a non-mobile baby may be associated with non-accidental impact head injury and are indicative of being gripped by the legs and swung [20].

Cases are underestimated
The true incidence of NAHI from shaking is unknown and the above figures are likely to be an underestimation. Reasons for this include:
- a lower level of reporting of child physical abuse to child protection agencies than would be expected from local prevalence statistics[21];
- children who are clearly symptomatic are more likely to be referred to social services and police than milder cases, and some recover without coming to hospital[22, 23].

This last point is supported by social research in one London Borough indicating that
- 1 in 9 mothers of under-2s may have shaken their baby
- 2 in 9 mothers may have felt like shaking their baby.

Such a large population is in contrast to the hospital-identified cases.
- This is also an underestimation as it does not include male partners, the most frequent perpetrator in hospital cases, or baby sitters and other carers [24].

Accidental head injury: incidence
Accidental head injuries are said to be more common than NAHIs, possibly 10–15 times more so in children under 1 year[25].
- A one year audit of A&E attendance of children under 1 year in a children's hospital in Scotland found that a high rate, 55%, were due to accidents[26].
- Half of these were head injuries.
- Falls were the cause in 61% of the cases.

- Six cases were judged to be non-accidental, five having head injuries: a parietal skull fracture, an intracranial bleed and three minor head injuries.

However, statistics from the neurosurgery clinics of North America suggest that 20–25 % of early childhood traumatic brain injury may be inflicted and in 64% of infants less than 1 year old it is probably caused by abuse[27].

This indicates how difficult it is to know the real incidence of non-accidental head injury, but among all types of physical abuse in small children, it is the largest killer and, with accidents, the case for prevention is overwhelming.

Outcomes of head injury

 Q **Why might the outcomes of NAHI be more serious than those for accidents?**

Clinical outcomes
The outcomes for NAHI are worse in general than from head injuries by other causes, such as road traffic accidents or serious falls. It is speculated that this may be because abused children are not brought for medical attention until they have significant injuries with dramatic symptoms secondary to the hypoxic damage to the brain itself[28].
- About one third of the children with non-accidental head injury die.
- Some two thirds of survivors have a level of permanent disability with associated learning disabilities such as cerebral palsy, visual, speech and language problems, seizures, autistic trait, hyperactive or aggressive behaviour.
- Fewer than 10 to 15% of babies recover completely.
- In the Severnside study some of those who apparently recovered were showing indications of behaviour and learning difficulties at school age[29].

Economic outcomes
Apart form the immediate clinical care, there is a cost burden arising from social, health, education and legal services (such as criminal compensation) for years, if not for life, following baby head injuries. For example:
- 24% of the surviving children for whom data were available in the Severnside study had a statement of special educational needs, compared with only 2–4% in the normal population.

Addressing accidental and non-accidental head injuries together

Q **What is misleading about the term shaken baby syndrome?**

The use of the term shaken baby syndrome is not without controversy. It draws attention to extreme cases and a specific mode of injury, rather than the overall priority to protect a baby's head from injuries with multi-factorial causes.

The term itself does not include injuries from blunt instruments or impact. It assumes clinical confidence in cause and effect where there are breathing difficulties, despite some uncertainties[3,30]. Further, it is not always easy to distinguish accidental from non-accidental injuries, or neglect, as they share some common features.

A case has been made to address both types of injury together in terms of policy,[31] prevention and health promotion,[2,32] and risks [1]. Newberger [33] describes such cases as paediatric social illnesses.

The suggestion that infant homicide might be reduced through preventive methods of working in alliance with parents, in the same way that Sudden Infant Deaths and accidental deaths have successfully been reduced, is raised by Creighton[15] in a review of fatal child abuse.

Similar negative social characteristics are noted for all these groups: they tend to be
- young,
- poor,
- ill-educated,
- disadvantaged,
- the non-accidental cases are more impoverished.

Dubowitz et al[1] argue that, conceptually, non-accidental and accidental injuries are two ends of a spectrum of childhood trauma.

The Severnside study
One aim of the Severnside study referenced above was to review the potential for preventing head injuries in babies.
- This was a retrospective case series of 90 children with subdural haemorrhage (SDH) in Wales and South West England.
- The cases were children under two years of age admitted to hospital between 1992 and 1998 with an SDH.
- Anonymised information was collected from hospital, community and legal records.

- 65 cases were found to be due to non-accidental injury, 9 due to medical cause, 9 unconfirmed causes, and 7 due to road traffic accidents or witnessed falls.

Explanations demonstrated a general failure to protect a baby's head in an unsafe home environment and dangerous child management practices.

3 | RISKS AND PREVENTION

What do we know about risk? How relevant is knowledge of risk factors for prediction, prevention and promoting safer head care?

The information on what happens in NAHI cases comes mainly from admissions of guilt by a caregiver or is established during police, court and social services investigation. Although valuable, this may be an incomplete picture. The Severnside study had 19 confessions by perpetrator and 10 cases where guilt was established by a criminal court.

Those responsible for non-accidental injuries do not readily confess, unlike in accidents where the history is readily forthcoming and matches the clinical findings[34]. In the Severnside study there were cases of unexplained injuries and cases with a major discrepancy of carer explanation and a significant injury, or developmentally incompatible history.

If it is not known how an injury happened, it is more difficult to identify risk and work preventatively.

Limitations of using risk factors

Q **Why might a risk check list not be a reliable means of deciding priorities for prevention interventions?**

The purpose of identifying risk factors is to predict who will harm a baby's head so that resources can be prioritised.
- The limitations of this approach include knowing that many risk factors are similar for other child abuse, accidents and Sudden Infant Deaths[35].
- There are no specific tools to predict head injury.
- There are doubts about screening with 1 correct prediction for 35 innocent families mislabelled as potentially abusive in one health visitor trial[36,37].
- Many cases may be missed.

This raises the question of the ethical acceptability of screening. Peters and Barlow[38] found that instruments designed to predict child maltreatment during antenatal and post natal periods had limited accuracy, were difficult to apply and could be stigmatising.

National guidelines in Canada also advise against screening with risk factors because of the low prevalence of child abuse in the population resulting in poor prediction[39]. However they do advocate from good evidence that

- disadvantaged families should be targeted with a home visiting programme from the perinatal period through infancy to prevent child abuse and neglect.

Targeted or universal prevention?

 What are the dangers of using risk factors alone to assess the likelihood of injury?

There is a common sense assumption that the more risk factors found in one case the higher the risk. Checklists are sometimes used in this way to prioritise need. However, of the eight more frequently observed risk factors in the Severnside study

- no cases had all the risk factors,
- most had one or two,
- one third appeared to have none and nothing is known about risk in those cases.

It is a paradox of prevention that large numbers with the condition to be prevented have no risk factors. This is an argument for a universal approach to prevention.

Risks are not certainties
Understanding that case associated characteristics are warning signs only, since risks are not certainties, implies that prevention should be through a population-wide rather than a targeted approach.

Studies have not been done to ascertain the relationship between apparent risk and the event. For example, not all parents with drug problems abuse their children. But it is wise to retain an awareness of what is known about risks to guide extra vigilance.

Effectiveness of prevention
Despite an assumption that accidental and non-accidental injuries are preventable, there is no comprehensive theoretical position or evidence base for non-accidental injury prevention to inform practitioners[40].

The USA is ahead here with NAHI prevention programmes in either hospitals or homes[41–44]. Many programmes work on the belief that parents may not be aware of the dangers of shaking, of the fragility of

subdural veins or the degree of strength needed to cause fractures.

One USA hospital intervention involves brief parent education at the time of birth in hospital to both mother and father and the signing of a Commitment Statement to say this has been received, as well as having posters around the ward, leaflets and a video.

This model has been developed and evaluated[41] in the New York State Region. It claims a 47% reduction in cases of shaken baby over a 5.5 year study period in children under three years old.

However a major difference between the USA and UK is that 93% of the parents in the study had already heard that shaking a baby was dangerous, whereas there is no widespread use of this information in the UK.

The hospital based education aimed to remind people at the right time and there is now a state wide mandate in Pennsylvania to provide the program to all parents of newborn infants.

The effectiveness of parent education in home visiting has been demonstrated in the prevention of both accidental and non accidental injuries, although more research for the latter is needed in the UK[45].

In the UK Hodnett and Roberts[46] summarised from a systematic review that home visiting support for socially disadvantaged mothers had a significant effect on maternal and child functioning, including improvements in levels of child abuse and neglect.

In Europe the World Health Organisation estimates that for each 1 Euro spent on home visits and education of parents about child abuse, 19 Euros will be saved[47].

However, it is questionable whether changing knowledge alone is enough to influence health behaviour in the field of child abuse. Accident prevention research also suggests that this is a partial approach to prevention[48].

Accident prevention
The field of accidental injury prevention in childhood has developed in a more robust way than non-accidental injury prevention. In reviewing the success internationally, Hemmo-Lotem and Danon[49] conclude that among the strategies that are most effective, especially in combination, are

- education and publicity,
- safer environments,
- promoting public policy,

- empowerment,
- data collection, evaluation and research.

A National Children's Bureau[50] review on home visiting and childhood injury summarises that
- home visits can reduce the risk of accidental injuries in the home by around 26 per cent,
- home visits may encourage parents to reduce home hazards,
- evidence is unclear on whether the effectiveness of home visiting in reducing injuries varies when provided by professionals, semi-professionals or specially trained community volunteers.
- the evidence for effectiveness of home visiting comes from studies of families with low-income and/or in high-accident areas.

The evidence of the effectiveness of home visiting in reducing accidental injury among children from ante- and post-natal home visiting[51] was positive in a review of reviews. However, it was inconclusive for any impact on child abuse, mainly because of methodological difficulties in comparing research. It recommended an urgent need to develop the UK evidence base in this area.

Non-accidental injury prevention

There are studies outside the UK which document the effectiveness of home visiting programmes and early interventions in reducing the maltreatment of children[52–54]. There are some elements in these studies which are common to effective abuse prevention interventions. These are that
- parenting education is best integrated with multiple community support programmes to promote and maintain healthy development;
- evaluation of parenting education should be ongoing with the other components.

In these studies from outside the UK, early home visiting can reduce child maltreatment (including abuse and neglect) in high risk families by as much as a 40%.
- Professional home visitors may be more effective than trained paraprofessionals, but longer duration programs with trained paraprofessionals can also be effective.
- Longer duration programs have larger effects.
- High risk is defined as e.g. single or young mothers, low income households, families with low birth weight infants.
- Home visiting is defined as a programme that includes trained personnel such as nurses or social workers visiting parents and children in their home to convey information, and/or offer support/training during a child's first two years of life.

Home visits may start in pregnancy and continue beyond two years of age.

2 | Strategies for prevention

4 | ACTIVITY FOR PREVENTION

The Severnside findings on risk and prevention
This section presents an analysis of the negative characteristics associated with abuse cases from the Severnside study and suggests prevention strategies for everyday practice to improve the effectiveness of prevention.

Infant characteristics

Q What characteristics of infants might lead to shaking?

Issue: Young babies are most at risk, males more than females

FACT
Severnside study[2-6]:
- 40 males and 25 females were identified with non-accidental head injury
- age range at injury from 19 days to 23 months (mean age 5.2 months)
- 57 under 1 year of whom 48 (74%) were 6 months or under
- Other studies: babies under 6 months are most common age; more are male.

The youngest baby of 19 days had had a previous hospital admission with a weak arm. He was subsequently found to have had a fractured clavicle relating to that event aged less than 2 weeks old. He was shaken to stop him crying.

What you might do

Q In what ways can the dangers of head injury be explained to parents?

- There is an Information sheet to share with parents tucked in the back cover.
- Peri-natal parent and carer education on protecting a baby's head, especially by avoiding shaking injuries, can be included routinely.
- If assessment of the quality of parenting is done this must be at an early age. Age one year is too late.
- Explain about a baby's vulnerability to head injury and the consequences.

The following are suggested educational messages for use with parents when a professional assesses their level of understanding and need. There are sources of help in the Practice Tools and the list of Resources at the end of this Section.

> If you feel unable to cope at any time, there are people who can help you. Asking for help or advice is a sign of good parenting.

> Shaking is dangerous. It causes brain damage because the neck muscles are weak and the joints in the neck are soft, like gristle, not like adult bone.

> The second neck bone has a protrusion that can wiggle about where it fits into the first neck bone. Strong movements of the head like shaking, or the impact of a bad fall, may cause internal bruising in the neck, which can spread up into the brain. This can interfere with the control of breathing, causing brain damage.

> Babies do not have a fully developed breathing system; it may easily be put under stress, causing lack of oxygen to the brain. This may lead to lifelong damage.

> If a baby is held by the chest and shaken the ribs may be compressed and broken.

> There are small delicate veins bridging a space between membranes that cover the brain. These may tear easily in a child as a result of force from shaking roughly, even for a short time, or an accident. It is thought that this may cause bleeding leading to brain damage from pressure in the head.

> Brain damage in babies has lasting effects like epilepsy, blindness, deafness and paralysis, as well as difficulties with behaviour and learning. It is also a cause of death.

Once brain damage has happened there is no going back. It cannot be undone.

Parent Information

Issue: A Parent Information leaflet is tucked in the back cover. It is designed to be accessible for those with low literacy ability.

FACT
Parents and health visitors have approved the following approach

What you might do

- The Parent Information can be photocopied
- The points can be shared with parents, explaining anything that is hard to understand, and discussing issues that arise.
- The leaflet can then be inserted in the Parent Held Child Record Book, or similar, and left for further reference.
- Points can be reinforced on future occasions. The use of the Child Accident Prevention home safety booklet 'I am only a baby but' reinforces the accident prevention messages (see Resources).

Information for fathers

Issue: It is vital that the information for parents is shared with fathers and other male carers

FACT
Males are the perpetrators of NAHI in more than 70% of cases.

What you might do

- If male carers are not available, mothers can be asked to show and discuss the information with them
- It is wise to check this has been done and record it.
- The websites on the Parent Information sheet may interest some fathers. Perhaps they can add other parenting websites to update the list?

Reasons given by parents for shaking

Issue: situations where a parent may feel out of control such as the baby having persistent crying, refusing to feed or won't stop fretting.

FACT
A Netherlands study of detrimental parent actions induced by infant crying in 3259 infants aged 1–6 months found that:
- At 6 months 5.6% of parents reported smothering, shaking or slapping (3.35% shaking)
- The crying may be of a normal nature and still provoke an abnormal and violent response. Parents may judge the crying as excessive and it is this perception that is significant[55].

What you might do
Parents can be educated about normal crying and how to cope. The following is a guide only. A baby should always be checked for signs of unwellness if crying persistently.

- The average one month old baby cries 1.5 hours per day but there is wide individual variation.
- Crying may peak at six weeks and decline by three months.
- Medically, excessive crying is defined as crying that lasts at least 3 hours a day, for 3 days a week, for at least 3 weeks.

- It is wise to be wary of adult behaviours that show lack of impulse control and empathy.
- Ask parents if they are worried about the baby's crying. Document the response and check at routine visits.
- If relevant, offer sources of help. If these are not available locally, inform service managers of need in writing.
- Do the same with parent concerns about feeding. Target the more complex parenting difficulties and refer appropriately.

Examples of sources of help:

Cry-sis
Helpline for parents with crying and sleepless children 020 7404 5011
7 day helpline open 8.0am–11.0pm

NSPCC Child Protection Helpline
Free, 24-hour service for anyone concerned about the safety of a baby or child
Telephone 0808 800 5000
Text phone 0800 056 0566

Parent and caregiver

 What might be some of the predisposing risk factors for non-accidental head injury?

Issue: who are the perpetrators?

FACTS FROM THE SEVERNSIDE STUDY
Parents
- 70% of abusers were male, in other studies 60%-90% of abusers were male, usually baby's father or mother's boyfriend
- Perpetrators were mainly in 2-parent families and were natural parents. 69% of mothers were living with the baby's father, 26 cohabiting and 19 married to father.

Social status
- Perpetrators were mostly of low socio-economic status but there were 3 parents of professional status and 6 college students out of the 65 abuse cases.
- Mother's average age was 23 years. The national average for first baby is nearer 30 years. There were 12/65 teenage parents but other studies show more.

Violence
- There was a history of violence in the relationship or criminal conviction in 40% of cases; other studies have similar rates.
- History of alcohol and or drug abuse, non-violent crime, mental illness including post natal depression, of being abused and or being in care as a child existed in 18%-26% of cases

Cases with no known risk factors
- One third of cases, 31%, appeared to have none of these negative characteristics. This means that they are valuable as pointers to raise awareness of the potential for abuse
Remember that abuse cases without common risk factors do occur.

What you might do

FATHERS AND MALE CARERS
- Involve fathers routinely in all discussion and education about protecting babies' heads from the earliest opportunity.
- Discuss in a professional forum how this can be achieved.
- Nominate a representative to liaise with Fathers Direct to see what is happening elsewhere
- Attend a conference, or take training in working with fathers and cascade this to your group.
- Have copies of a magazine for fathers in clinics.
- Advertise websites for fathers. For example:

Young Dads
A website aimed at young first-time fathers to answer questions they may be too embarrassed or intimidated to ask midwives
www.youngdads.co.uk

Fathers Direct
Online magazine for fathers and fathers-to-be
www.fathersdirect.com
Fathers Direct have developed national quality standards for father-friendly services. They have published a guide "Working with Fathers", designed to support staff working in family services who want to become more accessible to fathers, such as Sure Start, Early Years settings and maternity services.

What you might do: violence

 What negative feelings may parents and carers experience?

- Enquire about feelings and responses to baby behaviour. Negative feelings of anger and frustration have been reported.
- Document your observations.
- Do parents know that leaving the baby in the care of someone capable of violent behaviour is risky?

It has been hypothesised that the need to maintain control is the trigger to violent action, not that the person was violent by nature. Or perhaps perpetrators are lacking the interpersonal strategies for reducing danger in interfamilial situations and achieving comfort for themselves and others.
- What local resources are there for referral and help if violence is an issue?

What you might do: substance abuse

- Alert agencies managing cases of drug or alcohol abuse to the fact that there are children, especially babies, involved and to take this most vulnerable group into account with risk assessments.
- Document what has been done and for whom for prevention.

A list of risks has to be put in context. For example, how much of a risk a carer is with drug abuse depends on the severity of the abuse and how this affects the family lifestyle. There are 2 -3 million children in England and Wales with one or both parents having serious drug problems i.e. 2–3% of children under 16 years old[56].

Additional Risks: home environment

 Q Perpetrators of non-accidental and accidental head injury often have associated environmental risk factors. What might these include?

Issue: home safety

FACT

Descriptors of situations leading up to the injuries in the Severnside study included a catalogue of poor home safety, neglect, rough play, faulty treatment for choking, falls and dropping the baby.
The accidents in children under one in a hospital A&E audit found a similar cause of falls as explanations for accidents[26].

What you might do

- Assess the risks in the home environment for accidents.
- Look at local statistics on accidents to see if the neighbourhood is of high risk.
- Ask about home safety practices to modify risks by hazard removal, use of safety devices, supervision and modification of own behaviour.
- Suggest that head injury can be avoided by taking care with nursery equipment.
- Advise that older children should be supervised when handling a baby.
Incorporate these observations into a risk profile for the need to protect a baby's head to discuss with the family.

Additional Risks: past medical history

 Q What is the significance of the baby's past medical history when assessing the likelihood of abuse from shaking?

Issue: NAHI cases in the Severnside study had contact with health care professionals in the community and with hospital admissions prior to a diagnosis of non-accidental head injury.

FACT
- 74% (48/65) had contact with health professionals prior to diagnosis (excluding routine contacts)

HOSPITAL CONTACTS
- 48% (31/65) had been admitted to hospital
- 87% of these (27/31) had symptoms in retrospect relevant to a diagnosis of abuse from shaking, including fractures and bruises
- 29% (9/31) had been admitted more than once, 1–4 times

COMMUNITY CONTACTS
40% (26/65) of babies had been seen by a GP or health visitor 1–14 times (other than routine)
- Each had 1–3 symptoms in retrospect relevant to a diagnosis of abuse from shaking.
- Examples of babies seen by GP 4, 6, 10 and 14 times, the latter a 3 month old baby.

What you might do

- Ask about physical illness, visits to the doctor or hospital.
- Have an open mind and consider 'has this baby been shaken?'
- Might these frequent attendances be a cry for help?

Additional Risks: failure to protect a baby's head?

Issue: explanations given by parent or carer

FACT: TYPICAL HISTORIES IN THE SEVERNSIDE STUDY INCLUDED:

- baby being found unwell, having a fit and vomiting;
- histories of feeding problems and/or persistent crying;
- a history of bruising and fractures;
- having a fall, including being dropped, falling off a raised surface, out of a baby seat, off a sofa, chair, bed, stairs;
- faulty nursery or domestic equipment;
- sibling involved in accident;
- shaking admitted;
- vigorous rough play;
- no explanation;
- treated by shaking (for resuscitation or choking).

What you might do

- Observe parents' beliefs about control over baby and protectiveness
- Ensure parents know the signs of head injury, that rough play is risky, care must be taken on stairs
- Give out safety advice routinely from the earliest days.
- Ensure any home emergency care advice given does not include shaking for choking or resuscitation.

Additional Risks: caregiver history

 What might the history given by the carer include in a case of NAHI ?

Examples of more than one explanation offered and sometimes stories changed

Case 1 Mother found baby quiet and pale. Father (drunk) with baby 2 days previously. Moses basket frame collapsed and baby fell out. Father, an alcoholic, did not know what he had done.
Case 2 Partner looking after baby who fell downstairs and had a fit. Fell down a step and bumped head 3 weeks ago. Partner took child out of high chair and shook 3 days ago because of temper tantrum.
Case 3 Unwell for 3 days, off feeds. Deteriorated day of admission with 2 fits, moribund on admission.
Case 4 Baby not feeding 2 days, had a fit. Father admitted shaking due to work stress; held baby, squeezed chest and shook.

Examples of admission history related to being unwell prior to diagnosis of SDH

Case 1 Admitted one week previously with a fit following a few days vomiting and feeding problems, similar presentation at diagnosing event
Case 2 Admitted 3 times previously: drowsy and febrile, 5 days later vomiting, irritable, LP blood stained, bruising to thigh, 2 days later LP blood stained
Case 3 Admitted at 9 weeks old with same symptoms having been unwell, floppy, limp for 2–3 weeks; another similar admission 1 week prior to diagnosis.

Examples of admission history related to bruising prior to diagnosis of SDH

Case 1 3 admissions: age 3 weeks bruising abdomen, jaw and chin, shoulder, tongue and thigh, put on CPR; 5 days before death admitted with vomiting, bruise, constipated; seen in OPD day of death with bruised frenum, sent home
Case 2 2 weeks prior fell off sofa, 1 week later convulsion, bruises to back
Case 3 Infected pinna, bruises under feet, NAI queried 1 month previously

Examples of admission history related to fractures prior to diagnosis of SDH

Case 1 4 admissions: floppy, fits; age 2 months, slipped in bath bumped cheek; at 4 months floppy episodes meningitis excluded; at 7 months UTI, painful leg, fractures diagnosed, sent home, readmitted and SDH diagnosed
Case 2 Fractured tibia at 14 months, no explanation, treated by orthopaedic team, not seen by paediatrician until admitted SDH

These case examples are from the Severnside Study. They include the following abbreviations:

SDH	subdural haemorrhage
LP	lumber puncture
CPR	Child Protection Register
OPD	Out Patient Department
NAI	non-accidental injury
UTI	upper respiratory tract infection

Past medical history

Issue: has this baby been shaken?
If there is no enquiry about recent accidents or incidents affecting the baby's head the information may not be tied into the illness presentation.
Any unexplained illness that could be of neurological origin should be considered in the context of **'has this baby been shaken?'**

FACT
In view of the repeated hospital contacts and previous abuse, it is clear that the head injury abuse was not a one off event but a product of being in an environment that lends itself to abuse and accident.

What you might do

- Listen for a changing story about why the baby is unwell, what happened and when and who was the carer. Maintain a high level of suspicion if there are discrepant features to the explanation.
- Advise parents that if they know their baby has had any injury to the head or neck including a fall or being shaken they must tell the doctor so that the right treatment can be given promptly. Delay makes things worse.

Abuse is a process, not always a one off event

- There appears to be a pattern of parenting responses to an infant that include shaking or impact injuries from the very earliest days.

Abuse becomes a process rather than an event with a spectrum of degrees of shaking and of damage to the head with unknown outcomes for minor incidents which do not come to the attention of health services. Prevention needs to address both ends of the spectrum.

General principles of prevention

 Q **Can you identify prevention activities that you do, however informal? How do you know the impact of what has been done?**

Issue: There are many opportunities for preventive interventions in the home and for secondary prevention in follow up visits.

FACT
- Professionals who have contact in the peri-natal period with parents and carers already play an important preventive role.
But this may be hidden care as there is often a failure to identify the client group being protected. To do this is an aid to evaluation and identifies the need for resources.

What you might do

- Record in medical or care notes strategies used for the purpose of prevention as part of effective practice.
- Use a flow chart of problem, intervention and outcome.
- Record concerns e.g. quotes of negative comments by a parent about a baby, or concerns about the baby's physical health.
- Use a body map for any injury or bruise, however minor.
- Aggregate and share information with colleagues who may have contact with the family (the jigsaw approach).
This leads to visible outcomes and patterns of strategies to show what does or does not work.

Observe parenting capacity
Adding another dimension to the risk profile of observing parent/infant interaction to assess parenting capacity might improve the assessment [36].

Observations could be made and recorded at all early contacts of:
- the frequency of the parents' positive and negative statements about the infant and to the infant;
- the realistic perceptions of parents;
- the supportive, accessible and accepting parent behaviour.

Community focus: leaflets, posters, stickers to put on buggies or cots and videos. These are widely used in USA to target new parents in hospital, places where fathers meet, ante natal groups and adolescents in schools and clubs.

Work within your professional forum to learn where new knowledge can improve prevention. For example:

- Vulnerability indices are of doubtful use, but vulnerability assessments are more useful.
- Use a paper for discussion such as Vulnerability, need and significant harm: an analysis tool[57].

Protective factors

 What might the protective factors be in preventing injury to babies' heads?

How do people who are not neglectful protect a baby's head? What stops someone from shaking a baby? In the social study described earlier mothers who only felt like shaking their babies had had more contact with professionals. Is this a preventive factor? Feeling like and actually doing are different and we need to understand these differences and explain them to parents and carers.

Issue: Resilience factors
There is a theory, from mental health, that there are resilience factors or mitigating circumstances that protect from abuse, despite risk factors being present[58].

FACT
- Children vary in their vulnerability
- Multiple risk and protective factors are involved
- The aim is to reduce negative and increase positive factors
- Recognise how different risk factors interact
- Appreciate the role of peer group and community.
There are attributes in relationships that are thought to be protective and questions can be asked about parent and carer's general connectedness to others, compared with social isolation.

What you might do

Ask about attachment: friends, relatives, neighbourhood groups, established relationships with a professional person or mentor.
Observe what parents and carers do to protect the baby's head and pass these observations on to other parents.

5 | CONCLUSION AND KEY MESSAGES

A practice guide of the following points is tucked inside the back cover. This can be photocopied for use as an aide-mémoire. It has been designed at the request of health visitors to carry in their Diaries for everyday work.

Summary of preventive strategies

Stage 1: Information gathering
- Evaluate what parents know about risk of head injury
- Evaluate the environment and social characteristics
- Enquire about the past medical history
- Evaluate what is known about protective factors

Stage 2: Strategies for prevention
- Ante-natal visits are the first opportunity to assess and educate
- Aim to reduce the negative risk factors and build the positive protective ones
- Educate about the realities of parenting like coping with crying babies
- Use the benefit of support groups like post natal depression and domestic conflict and violence
- Practice continuity of care and inter-professional collaboration.

Dimensions of a risk check for accidental and non-accidental injury

- **Peri-natal:** young babies are most at risk. Give prevention information at earliest contact like antenatal visits.
- **Social factors:** not all cases have the known risks but vigilance is raised where there is violence, mental illness, substance abuse, criminal conviction, and previous abuse.
- **Environmental factors:** unsafe homes and a failure to protect the baby's head. Promote a learning zone of safe handling and protecting babies' heads.
- **Parenting capacity** has strong associations with socio-economic deprivation. Assess support and attachments.
- **Medical events** and signs of abuse: where minor, isolated neurological events and bruising are observed with repeat hospital admissions.

6 | REFERENCES key papers are highlighted

1 Dubowitz H, Hampton RL, Bithoney WG, Newberger EH. Inflicted and non inflicted injuries: differences in child and familial characteristics. Am J Orthopsychiatry 1987 Oct; 57(4):525–35.

2 Coles L, Kemp AM. Cues and clues to preventing shaken baby syndrome. Community Practitioner 2003; 76(12): 459–463.

3 Kemp AM, Stoodley N, Cobley C, Coles L, Kemp K. Apnoea and brain swelling in non-accidental head injury. *Archives of Disease Childhood* 2003; 88:472–476.

4 Kemp AM, Coles L. The role of health professionals in preventing non-accidental head injury. *Child Abuse Review* 2003; 12(6): 374–383.

5 Sanders T, Cobley C, Coles L, Kemp AM. Factors affecting referral of young children with severe head injury to child protection agencies: a case series. *Child Abuse Review* 2003; 12(6): 358–373.

6 Kemp AM. Investigating subdural haemorrhage in infants. *Archives of Disease in Childhood* 2002; 86(2): 98–102.

7 DfES. *Every Child Matters* London: Stationary Office; 2004.

8 Wanless, Derek (author of *Securing Our Future Health: Taking a Long Term View* DoH) Advisor to the *Review of Health and Social Care in Wales.* Cardiff; Welsh Assembly Government; 2003.

9 Lord Laming. *Inquiry into the death of Victoria Climbié.* London: Stationery Office; 2003.

10 Hall D. Child protection – lessons from Victoria Climbié. *BMJ* 2003 326:293–4.

11 Duhaime AC, Christian CW, Rorke LR, Zimmerman RA. Non-accidental head trauma in infants-the "shaken baby syndrome". N Engl J Med 1999; 338:1822–1829.

12 Barlow KM, Minns RA. Annual incidence of shaken impact syndrome in young children. Lancet 2000; 356;1571–1572.

13 Jayawant S, Rawlinson A, Gibbon F, Price J, Schulte J, Sharples P, Sibert J, Kemp AM. Subdural haemorrhages in infants: population based study. BMJ 1998 317;1558–1561.

14 Health Statistics Quarterly. Autumn 2003 http://www.statistics.gov.uk

15 Creighton SJ. Fatal Child Abuse-How Preventable is it? Child Abuse Review 1995; 4: 318–328.

16 HOWIS The Health of Wales Information Service. http://www.wales.nhs.uk

17 Sibert JR, Payne EH, Kemp AM, Barber M, Rolfe K, Morgan RJH, Lyons RA, Butler I. The incidence of severe physical abuse in Wales. Child Abuse and Neglect 2002; 26: 267–276.

18 Guthkelch AN. Infantile subdural haematoma and its relationship to whiplash injury BMJ 1971; 2:430–1.

19 Caffey J. On the theory and practice of shaking infants: its potential residual effects of permanent brain damage and mental retardation. American Journal of Diseases in Childhood 1972 124: 161–9.

20 Atwal GS, Rutty G.N, Carter N, Green MA. Bruising in non-accidental head injured children; a retrospective study of the prevalence, distribution and pathological associations in 24 cases. Forensic Science International 1998; 96: 215–230.

21 Sidebotham PD. Audit of child protection procedures in accident and emergency department to identify children at risk of abuse. BMJ 1997; 315: 855–856.

22 Jenny C, Hymel KP, Ritzen A, Reinert SE, Hay TC. Analysis of missed cases of abusive head trauma. Journal of the American Medical Association 1999; 282: 621–626.

23 Morris JL, Johnson CF, Clasen M. To report or not to report: physicians' attitudes towards discipline and child abuse. American Journal of Diseases of Children 1985; 139: 194–197.

24 Shepherd J, Sampson A. 'Don't Shake the Baby': towards a prevention strategy. British Journal of Social Work 2000; 30,721–735.

25 Claydon SM. Fatal extradural haemorrhage following a fall from a baby bouncer. Pediatr Emerg Care 1996; 12: 432–4.

26 Magregor DM. Accident and emergency attendances by children under the age of 1 year as a result of injury. Emerg Med J 2003; 20:21–24.

27 Beers SR, De Bellis MD. Outcomes of child abuse. Neurosurgery Clinics of North America 2002; 13 (2):235–241.

28 Bechtel K, Stoessel K, Leventhal JM, Ogle E, Teague B, Lavietes S, Banyas B, Allen K, Dziura J, Duncan C. Characteristics that distinguish accidental from abusive injury in hospitalized young children with head trauma. Pediatrics 2004 Jul;114(1):165–8.

29 Karandikar S, Coles L, Jayawant S, Kemp AM. Neurodevelopmental outcome in shaken baby syndrome *Child Abuse Review* 2004; 13(3): 178–187.

30 Geddes JF, Hackshaw AK, Vowles GH, Nickols CD, Whitwell HL. Neuropathology of inflicted head injury in children (1 Patterns of brain injury). Brain 2001; 124(7): 1290–1298.

31 Thompson AH, Borden K, Belton KL. Intentional and unintentional injuries across health regions in Alberta, Canada: an implication for policy. Crisis 2004; 25(4): 156–60.

32 Tomashek KM, Hsia J, Iyasu S. Trends in postneonatal mortality attributable to injury, United States 1988–1998. Paediatrics 2003 111; 5: 1219–1225.

33 Newberger EH, Hampton RL, Marx TJ, White K. Child abuse and pediatric social illness: an epidemiological analysis and ecological reformulation. Amer J Orthopsychiat 1986; 56(4) 589–601.

34 Hettler J, Greenes D. Can the initial history predict whether a child with head injury has been abused? Pediatrics 2003; 11(3): 602–607.

35 Fleming PJ, Blair PS, Ward Platt M, Tripp J, Smith, IJ. Sudden infant death syndrome and social deprivation: assessing epidemiological factors after post-matching for deprivation. Paediatric & Perinatal Epidemiology 2003; 17 (3), 272–280.

36 Browne K, Hanks H, Stratton P, Hamilton C Editors. Early Prediction and Prevention of Child Abuse. Chichester: Wiley; 2002.

37 Barker W. Practical and ethical doubts about screening for child abuse. Health Visitor 1990; 63(1): 14–17.

38 Peters R, Barlow J. Systematic Review of Instruments Designed to Predict Child Maltreatment During the Antenatal and Postnatal periods. Child Abuse Review 2003; 12:416–439.

39 MacMillan HL. Preventive health care 2000 update: prevention of child maltreatment, Canadian Centre for Studies of Children at Risk, McMaster University, Hamilton, Ontario. CMAJ 2000 Nov 28; 163(11):1451–8.

40 Davies WH, Garwood MM. Who are the perpetrators and why do they do it? (Shaken Baby Syndrome). Journal of Aggression, Maltreatment and Trauma 2001; 5(1): 41–45.

41 Dias MS, Smith K, deGuehery K, Mazur P, Li Veetai, Shaffer ML. Preventing Abusive Head Trauma Among Infants and Young Children: A Hospital-Based, Parent Education Program. Pediatrics 2005; 115;470–477.

42 Olds D, Henderson C, Eckenrode J. Preventing child abuse and neglect with prenatal and infancy home visiting by nurses. In: Browne K, Hanks H, Stratton P, Hamilton C, editors. Early Prediction and Prevention of Child Abuse. Wiley: Chichester; 2002 p.165 -183.

43 Showers J. Preventing Shaken Baby Syndrome. Journal of Aggression, Maltreatment and Trauma 2001; 5(1): 349–365.

44 Olds D, Henderson CRJ, Kitzman H, Cole R. Effects of prenatal and infancy nurse home visitation on surveillance of child maltreatment. Pediatrics 1995; 95: 365–372.

45 Roberts I, Kramer MS, Suissa S. Does home visiting prevent childhood injury? A systematic review of randomised controlled trials. BMJ 1996; 312:29–33.

46 Hodnett ED, Roberts I. Home-based social support for socially disadvantaged mothers. Cochrane database Syst Rev 2000;(2):CD000107.

47 World Health Organisation. The solid facts on unintentional injuries and violence in the WHO European Region. Fact sheet Euro/11/05 Copenhagen, Bucharest, 12 September 2005.

48 Assum T. Attitudes and road accident risk. Accid Anal Prev 1997; 29(2):153–9.

49 Hemmo-Lotem M, Danon Y. Childhood injuries in Israel: status and prevention strategies. Harefuah 2003 Sep; 142(8–9):609–11, 646, 645.

50 National Children's Bureau. Highlight no 213 Library and Information Services 2004 www.ncb.org.uk 8 Wakley Street, London EC1V 7QE.

51 Bull J, McCormick G, Swann C, Mulvihill C. Ante- and post-natal home visiting programmes: a review of reviews. London: HDA; 2004.

52 Geeraert L, Van den Noortgate L, Grietens H, Onghena P. The effects of early prevention programs for families with young children at risk of physical child abuse and neglect: a meta analysis. Child Maltreatment 2004; 9(3): 277–291.

53 World Health Organisation. Child abuse and neglect by parents and caregivers In: World Report on Violence and Health. WHO: Geneva; 2002 Chapter 3

54 Centres for Disease Control and Prevention. First Reports Evaluating the Effectiveness of strategies for preventing Violence: Early Childhood Home Visitation and Firearms Laws. Findings from the Task Force on Community Preventive Services. MMWR 2003; 52(RR-14)

55 Reijneveld SA et al. Infant crying and abuse Lancet. 2004 Oct 9; 364: 1340–42.

56 Home Office. Executive summary. In: Hidden Harm: Inquiry by the Advisory Council on the Misuse of Drugs-Prevention working group. London: Stationery Office; 2004. www.drugs.gov.uk

57 Scott L. Vulnerability, need and significant harm: an analysis tool. Community Practitioner 2003; 76(12): 468–473.

58 Rutter M. Resilience concepts and findings: implications for family therapy. Journal of Family Therapy 1999; 21(2): 119–144.

RESOURCES AND WEBSITES

Suzanne Franklin Carbaugh. Understanding shaken baby syndrome. Advances in Neonatal Care 2004 April; 4(2) 105–117.

Suzanne Franklin Carbaugh. Preventing shaken baby syndrome: Family teaching toolbox. Advances in Neonatal Care 2004 April; 4(2) 118–119.

Preventing child abuse
NSPCC Child Protection Helpline
Free, 24-hour service for anyone concerned about the safety of a baby or child
Telephone 0808 800 5000
Text phone 0800 056 0566
http://www.nspcc.org.uk

Preventing Child Abuse & Neglect (USA)
Resources to help parents and communities understand and meet children's needs and protect them from harm. Includes information on child abuse and neglect prevention, risk and protective factors, recognizing and reporting abuse, family support, positive parenting, prevention programs, public awareness.
www.childwelfare.gov/preventing

Shaken baby syndrome
http://www.dontshake.com (USA)

Working with fathers
www.fathersdirect.com (UK Father Pack)
www.youngdads.co.uk
www.children-ne.org (Children North East/Fathers Plus)

The Importance of Fathers in the Healthy Development of Children (USA).
http://www.childwelfare.gov/pubs/usermanuals/fatherhood

Support for crying babies
Cry-Sis Helpline 08451 228 669
http://www.cry-sis.org.uk

Coping with crying babies. Leaflet
http://www.nspcc.org.uk
NSPCC Helpline 0808 800 5000

Accident prevention
Child Accident Prevention Trust 020 7608 3828
Accident prevention booklet I am only a baby but.
http://www.capt.org.uk

Parenting
Parentline Plus (UK)
A national charity offering help and information for parents, carers and families via a range of services including a free 24hr confidential helpline, workshops, courses, information leaflets, email and website
http://www.parentlineplus.org.uk
Helpline: 0808 800 2222

The Parent Connection (One plus One) (UK)
For parents: This website has information and tips to help you to deal with things that may affect your relationship and also other sources of information and support. The Parent Connection aims to encourage you to think about the importance of your relationship with your child's other parent, whether or not you are still together, and the impact this has on your child.
http://www.theparentconnection.org.uk

A_Z Parenting website (Australia)
Colourful, practical, age related website. Covers normal crying in newborns and information for Dads.
http://raisingchildren.net.au/